How Do I Write a Good Compare and Contrast Essay?
From Start to Finish
Essay Writing Success Series Volume 2

by

Julie Jones

© www.beststudentsuccessseries.com

To learn about the other books I have written which lead to better grades and study skills, click here
http://www.beststudentsuccessseries.com.

Copyright © 2015 J Rembrandt Int'l
All rights reserved. No part of this publication may be reproduced, stored in a retrieval system, or transmitted in any form, or by any means, electronic, mechanical, photocopying, recording or otherwise, without prior consent of the publisher. Printed in the United States.
ISBN:
ISBN-13: 978-0-9842493-7-4
ISBN-10: 0-9842493-7-0
eISBN-13: 978-0-9842493-8-1
eISBN-10: 0-9842493-8-9

© www.beststudentsuccessseries.com

DEDICATION

I love you, Victor, my son. You will never know how much I love you and appreciate your help.

MY OTHER BOOKS

Vocabulary to teach kids: 30 days to increased vocabulary and improved reading comprehension (best student success series book 1) - This book is good for ages 8 and up. It is best for teens 12 – 22.

How Do I Write a Good Explanatory Essay? From Start to Finish (Essay Writing Success Series Volume 1) - This book is good for ages 8 and up. It is best for teens 12 – 22.

© http://www.beststudentsuccessseries.com

Table of Contents

Start Here 7
Thank you 8
Who is this book for? 8
How is this book designed? 8
Let's Get Started 8
Review – Important Terms to Remember 11
Review – the Essentials of Writing 13
How do I understand a writing prompt? 19
Why is it important that I pre-write or brainstorm in preparation of writing my 5 paragraph explanatory essay? 25
How do I write an outline for my 5 paragraph explanatory essay? 29
How do I write my 5 paragraph explanatory essay? 35
Lessons Learned 41
Appendix A - Transition Words 43

PAGE LEFT BLANK INTENTIONALLY

Start Here

Thank you

Before we begin, I want to thank you for buying my book. I wrote this book because I found it very difficult to find a way to improve my writing and my son's writing after years of research for the right materials, I finally found a way to improve our writing. I wrote this to prevent you from having to suffer through years of research on how to improve your writing or your child's writing. I have done all the work for you. This is written in a clear concise manner so you can learn to write a 5 paragraph explanatory essay and move on with your life. If you find this book helpful, I need **your help**. Please do the following:
1) **tell** your friends and family to **buy** my book
2) **leave positive feedback** on Amazon.com
3) **visit** my website which is www.beststudentsuccessseries.com to find other books I have written as well as other resources.

Who is this book for?

This book is for 10-to-22-year-olds or anyone who wants to know how to write a 5 paragraph explanatory or informative essay especially for the common core or **any** standardized test. It will also make classroom assignments and any homework writing assignments much easier.

How is this book designed?

This book is designed to help you understand how to identify when the writing prompt or assignment requires an explanatory essay, then explains how to write the explanatory essay from start to finish. The chapters are as follows:

1. Review – the Essentials of Writing
2. How to understand a writing prompt
3. Why you should pre-write your essay
4. How to write your outline
5. How to write your essay

After reading this book, you will know how to write a focused, clear and concise 5 paragraph explanatory or informative essay.

Let's Get Started

This book is 43 pages. You and your child should read the entire book together first. Try to do this in 3 days or less. Just to make sure you both understand everything first. Then, have your child go back to read everything and complete all instructions. Do this in 30 days or less to get the most benefits from the book. To make sure you and your child get everything done in 30 days or less, make sure you mark your calendar for each day you are going to complete an assignment.

PAGE LEFT BLANK INTENTIONALLY

Review – Important Terms to Remember

Here we are going to review important terms to when writing an essay. Some of the words you are already familiar with. It is important to know these terms because I will discuss them in the book and I want to be sure that you have clear understanding of the words mean so that when I explain how to create them for your essay you know what they mean.

What is a **5 paragraph essay**? In the book, I will mention 5 paragraph essay a lot because it's usually at least one written page or typed page in length. This is important because it give a gauge or rule of thumb on how much information you must put into an assignment.

What is an **introduction** to an essay? The purpose of writing an introduction to an essay is to inform the reader what he/ she will learn while reading the essay while including the answers to the writing prompt.

What is a **body paragraph**? A body paragraph has its own main topic sentence and at 3 supporting detail sentences and supports or refers back to the main topic or question answered regarding the writing prompt.

What are **supporting details**? Supporting details of a paragraph explains the what, where, when, why and how of the main topic or question answered regarding the writing prompt.

What is a **conclusion**? A conclusion does 2 things:
   a) Restates the introduction of the essay in different words
   b) Informs the reader what he/ she should have learned in the essay

In conclusion, we will discuss these terms in full detail and actually learn the thought process you must have to create them later on in the book.

Review – the Essentials of Writing

In order for you to get a clear understanding of how to write a 5 paragraph explanatory essay, we must review the following first:
- Basic structure of a sentence
- Listing information or data in a series
- Using transition words
- Basic structure of a paragraph

Understanding how to write at the most basic level will help you as your writing advances because you understand it at its most basic level.

Remember this book gives you the opportunity to get comfortable through practice with writing a 5 paragraph explanatory essay so pay close attention the examples because you will be expected to write or type your own examples as practice or write or type the examples provided as practice. Also, when you get to the review section make sure you write down your answer whether it is in a separate notebook or in this book.

Basic structure of a sentence

According to www.oxforddictionaries.com, a sentence is a set of words that is complete in itself, typically containing a subject and predicate, conveying a statement, question, exclamation, or command, and consisting of a main clause and sometimes one or more subordinate clauses.

A simpler way to look at is a sentence has a subject which is a noun and a predicate which completes the sentence. If you generally speak English without slang, chances are you are probably speaking in complete sentences.

For example, look at the following sentence:

I can ride a bike.

I is the subject or the noun. Can and ride are verbs. Bike is a noun. Another way to look at is, the words *can ride a bike* is a predicate. This is not an in depth explanation of sentence structure, but I just want you to understand the basic structure of a sentence.

Listing information or data in a series

When you have to explain two or more things in writing, it is helpful to write the list in a series.

For instance, if I am writing a list of the following fruits:
- Apple
- Pear
- Grape

If I need to explain in a paragraph, I will list it in a series as follows:

apple, pear and grapes

Notice the comma separating each fruit or item. Then, you need to put the word '**and**' before the last word or item.

Now that you see how a series looks, let's look at it as it relates to listing details you are going to write about in a paragraph. We are going to discuss an explanatory essay on how to ride a bike in the following chapters so consider the following list:

- Balance yourself on the bike
- Balance yourself and pedal while on the bike
- Learn how to stop the bike

If I need to explain in a paragraph, I will list it in a series in my introductory paragraph as follows:

balance yourself on the bike, balance yourself and pedal while on the bike, and learn how to stop the bike

Do you understand how to make a list in a series? Circle one. **Yes** or **No**. You will need to know this information in order to list what you are going to write about in a paragraph in a series.

Using transition words

What is a transition word? When you move from paragraph to paragraph a transition word helps with the flow from paragraph to paragraph by making it sound like the paragraphs are connected. (See the **Appendix A**. for a list of transition words) A transition word will start each of your 3 body paragraphs.

There are many examples of transition words, but here are the most basic ones that you can't go wrong with using:

1. first, second, third
2. first, next, last

We are going to use these words when you write our 5 paragraph explanatory essay.

Basic structure of a paragraph

There 5 parts to the basic structure of a paragraph. They are the main topic sentence, 3 supporting detail sentences and a summary sentence.

What is a main topic sentence? It tells what the paragraph is about.

What is a supporting detail? It gives details to support the main topic sentence.

© http://www.beststudentsuccessseries.com

What is a summary sentence? A summary sentence gives a summary of what the paragraph was about.

There 3 steps to riding a bicycle. **First**, you must learn how to balance yourself on the bike. **Second**, you must learn how to pedal while balancing yourself on the bike. **Third**, you must learn how to stop on the bike. Riding a bike seems easy, but it is hard to learn. However, once you learn you never forget how to ride a bike.

There 3 steps to riding a bicycle. **Here is the main topic sentence.**

Here are the 3 supporting detail sentences:

First, you must learn how to balance yourself on the bike. **Second**, you must learn how to pedal while balancing yourself on the bike. **Third**, you must learn how to stop on the bike.

Here are the summary sentences:

Riding a bike seems easy, but it is hard to learn. However, once you learn you never forget how to ride a bike.

In conclusion, this review of the essentials of writing is designed to help you understand writing at its most basic level so that you can improve your writing. Did this review help you? Do you see anything that can help you improve your writing? You will need a clear understanding of these concepts if you expect to learn how to write a 5 paragraph explanatory essay.

Summary:

Please answer the following questions:
Do you know understand the basic structure of a sentence?
Do you understand how to write a list of 3 or more items in a series?
Do you know what transition words are?
Do you know a few words that you can use as transitions?
Do you understand the structure of a paragraph?

If you answered, *no* to any one of the above questions, then re-read the entire chapter until you can answer yes to each of the above questions. Why? Because it will help build your knowledge so that when you are faced with the situation of writing an explanatory essay, you will know what to do.

If you answered, *yes* to all of the above questions, then we can proceed because you have an action plan in mind of how to write a 5 paragraph explanatory essay. At the end of the chapter, I will review your knowledge. You can use the information in this chapter to answer the questions so it is open-book, but *you* **must** **write your answers down**.

Takeaways:
1) This is an example of writing information in a series:
   - balance yourself on the bike, balance yourself and pedal while on the bike, and learn how to stop the bike
2) This is an example of writing items in a series:
   - apple, pear and grapes
3) By using the following words to transition from by body paragraph to body paragraph, it will help the flow of your essay or paragraph:
   - First
   - Second
   - Third
4) A paragraph must have the following 5 types of sentences to be complete:
   - a main topic sentence or paragraph
   - 3 supporting detail sentences
   - concluding/ summary sentence

Review:

Please answer the following questions *in writing or by typing*:

- What 3 words can you use to transition from each of your 3 body paragraphs?
- How do you list 3 or more items in a series?
- Give an example of a basic sentence?
- What 3 things a basic paragraph must have?

© http://www.beststudentsuccessseries.com

PAGE LEFT BLANK INTENTIONALLY

How do I understand a writing prompt?

Before we get started with understanding a compare and contrast writing prompt, I want you to download your free gift.

Your Free Gift

As a way of saying *thank you* to my readers and to show you how committed I'm to making sure that you learn how to write a compare and contrast essay, I am giving you FREE access to my compare and contrast essay outline (value $19.99)

It will help you **understand** how to write a compare and contrast essay **easily** and **quickly**. It is designed as companion to this book so I recommend that you use it while reading the book.
http://www.beststudentsuccessseries.com/essay-template/

http://www.beststudentsuccessseries.com/essay-template/

In this chapter, I am going to show you how to understand a writing prompt. Understanding a writing prompt is important because it determines how you focus your writing. I am going to show you a writing prompt, define a compare and contrast essay, tell you what key words to look for and how to determine what information you need to put in your essay.

Here is the writing prompt we are going to discuss:

Writing Situation

Think about an apple and an orange.

Writing Task

Write a 5 paragraph essay to compare and contrast an apple and an orange.

What is a compare and contrast essay? A compare and contrast essay is meant to inform the reader the similarities (compare) and the differences (contrast) between 2 things or subjects (i.e., objects, events, people, theme of books or places)—closely related or vastly different—and focuses on what about them is the same or what's different or focuses on a combination of similarities and differences. The comparison between the two is to:

- State something unknown.

- Clear up a misunderstanding.
- Show that one thing is superior to another.
- Lead to a new way of doing/seeing/understanding something.
- Argue a point with supported facts.

Think of compare and contrast as a way to explain the similarities and the differences between two subjects in 5 paragraph.

Figure 1. Example of a list.
Similarities between an apple and an orange
1. Both are fruits
2. Both grow on trees
3. Both can be eaten peeled
4. There are different types of apples and oranges

Differences between an apple and an orange
1. Apple
    a. you can eat the skin
    b. Come in different colors
2. Orange
    a. You can only eat the skin if you grate it and use it as a zest in food
    b. Comes pre-sliced from nature

What do I do if I have to write about a topic that I am not interested in or don't know about? In this instance you must use your imagination to write the essay, but make it sound realistic or like something your supporting details could possibly happen. How? By drawing reference from things you have heard on the news, friend's stories, movies you have watched, these are just some examples.

How do I identify whether or not a writing prompt is of a compare and contrast essay? Sometimes the directions will explicitly state that you need to write a compare and contrast essay. When it is not stated you will need to look for key words such as similarities and differences between something.

For example, in the writing prompt it says **compare** and **contrast** (see below) so in this case you need to compare and contrast an apple and an orange.

Writing Situation

Think about an apple and an orange.

Writing Task - Explained

Write a 5 paragraph essay to **compare** and **contrast** an apple and an orange.

How do I know what I need to focus my writing on? Some writing prompts have questions in them. In this case you would answer the question by turning the question or questions into a statement. In other instances, where what you need to focus your writing on is not so clear, then look for keywords in the writing prompt which **tells you to explain the similarities and differences between something** such as books, objects, situations, etc.

For example, this writing prompt says to compare and contrast an apple and an orange so I need to write a 5 paragraph essay comparing the similarities and the differences between an apple and an orange. To write it as a question, I would say:

What are the similarities and differences between an apple and an orange?
Also, if it is clear you want to know the purpose of comparing and contrasting the subjects such to show one superior to the other, to clear up a misunderstanding, etc. Otherwise, you should understand that you have to create your own purpose in the writing, in addition to compare and contrast.

In conclusion, when reading a writing prompt it is important to understand what type of essay you need to write, what questions you need to answer in your writing and the purpose. These are the *keys* to focused, clear and concise writing which leads to good grades.

Summary:

Please answer the following questions:
Do you know the purpose of writing a compare and contrast essay?

Do you know how to turn a compare and contrast essay writing prompt into a question?

Do you know what words you can look for to identify that the writing prompt is a compare and contrast essay?

Do you know what information you can use as references to write a compare and contrast essay if you are not familiar with the subject matter or don't like it?

If you answered, *no* to any one of the above questions, then re-read the entire chapter until you can answer yes to each of the above questions. Why? Because it will help build your knowledge so that when you are faced with the situation of writing a compare and contrast essay, you will know what to do.

If you answered, *yes* to all of the above questions, then we can proceed because you have an action plan in mind of how understand a compare and contrast essay writing prompt. At the end of the chapter, I will review your knowledge. You can use the

© http://www.beststudentsuccesssseries.com

information in this chapter to answer the questions so it is open-book, but **you must write your answers down**.

Takeaways:

1) A compare and contrast is meant to inform the reader how to do something real or imagined. If it is imagined, your writing must make sense like it is possible.
2) To identify whether a writing prompt is a compare and contrast essay when it is not stated explicitly, you need to look for the keywords such as similarities and differences, compare and contrast. etc.
3) By turning a compare and contrast essay into a question before you start writing, you will make your writing more focused and clear.

Review:

Please answer the following questions *in writing or by typing*:

- What can you turn your writing prompt into to make it easier to answer?
- What is the purpose of a compare and contrast essay?
- What key words can you look for in the writing prompt to identify that it is for a
- compare and contrast essay?
- What can you use as references to help improve your writing if you are writing about a subject you are not familiar with or don't know about?

PAGE LEFT BLANK INTENTIONALLY

Why is it important that I pre-write or brainstorm in preparation of writing my 5 paragraph compare and contrast essay?

In the previous chapter, I showed you how to understand and identify a compare and contrast essay writing prompt. Next, we are going to take about pre-writing or brainstorming for the same writing prompt. During this stage, it is very important that you write anything and everything you can think of without restriction because of the information will be useful and some will not be useful.

If you need a reminder of the writing prompt we are discussing, here it is again:

Writing Situation

Think about an apple and an orange.

Writing Task

Write a 5 paragraph essay to **compare** and **contrast** an apple and an orange.

What is pre-writing or brainstorming? Pre-writing or brainstorming is the process of writing down what first comes to your mind when you are reading the writing prompt without worrying about sequencing or whether or not it fits the assignment. Why is *writing down* what first comes to your mind **important**? There are two reasons:

1) It is easier to organize your thoughts when they are WRITTEN or typed which is very helpful when you are at the outline stage.
2) It is a good way to clear your mind and focus your writing

When pre-writing or brainstorming, you don't write complete sentences. You write just enough so that it triggers your memory about what you want to include in your essay because you want to write as much information down as you can so that you can move on to the next steps of refining your writing. Some of your pre-writing or brainstorming will be relevant and some of it will not be.

Pre-writing (**Hint:** Write the question or questions down that you need to answer in your essay.)

> **Question to answer with pre-writing or brainstorming:** What are the similarities and differences between an apple and an orange?
>
> Similarities between an apple and an orange
>   1. Both are fruits
>   2. Both grow on trees
>   3. Both can be eaten peeled
>   4. There are different types of apples and oranges
>
> Differences between an apple and an orange
>   1. Apple
>   a. you can eat the skin

        b. Come in different colors
    2. Orange
        a. You can only eat the skin if you grate it and use it as a zest in food
        b. Comes pre-sliced from nature

In my pre-writing or brainstorming, I came up with 4 similarities and 3 things that I can use to contrast an apple and an orange. Depending on how I write my essay this may be enough information, but I won't know until I complete my outline and do a first draft.

Just to recap. My **final** pre-writing or brainstorming is as follows:

What are the similarities and differences between an apple and an orange?

Similarities between an apple and an orange
1. Both are fruits
2. Both grow on trees
3. Both can be eaten peeled
4. There are different types of apples and oranges

Differences between an apple and an orange
1. Apple
    a. you can eat the skin
    b. Come in different colors
2. Orange
    a. You can only eat the skin if you grate it and use it as a zest in food
    b. Comes pre-sliced from nature

In conclusion, pre-writing or brainstorming is important to the writing process because it allows you get your thoughts down on paper where it is easier to analyze and organize. In other words, it is more difficult review and organize your thoughts without first writing them down or typing them.

Summary:

Please answer the following questions:
Do you know what pre-writing or brainstorming means?
Do you know why it is important to pre-write or brainstorm?

If you answered **no** to any one of the above questions, then re-read the entire chapter until you can answer yes to each of the above questions. Why? Because it will help build your knowledge so that when you are faced with the situation of writing an explanatory essay, you will know what to do.

If you answered, **yes** to all of the above questions, then we can proceed because you have an action plan in mind of how to pre-write or brainstorm an essay writing assignment. I will review your knowledge at the end of the chapter. You can use the information in this chapter to answer the questions so it is open-book, but *you* **must write your answers down**.

Takeaways:

1) Pre-writing or brainstorming is the process of writing down what first comes to your mind when you are reading the writing prompt without worrying about sequencing. To identify whether a writing prompt is a compare and contrast essay when it is not stated explicitly, you need to look for the keywords such as explain, discuss, similarities and differences, compare and contrast, etc.

2) Pre-writing or brainstorming is important because it helps you organize your thoughts and clears your mind so that you can focus your writing

Review:

Please answer the following questions in writing or by typing:

- What is pre-writing or brainstorming?
- Why is pre-writing or brainstorming important?

How do I write an outline for my 5 paragraph compare and contrast essay?

In the previous lesson, we learn how pre-writing or brainstorming can help you focus your writing. We are going to learn how to write an outline for your compare and contrast essay. By creating an outline that is reflective of a 5 paragraph essay with an introduction, 3 supporting detail and conclusion.

Outline

What is an outline? An outline gives a brief explanation of what you are going to write about in an essay or paragraph in list form. It doesn't have to be in complete sentences unless you have instructions otherwise.

Why is it important to write and outline? An outline helps you organize your thoughts in list form and helps you see what you are going to write about. If this doesn't make sense don't worry, you will understand better as you read more and review the examples that I have provided.

Introduction

What is an introduction? The purpose of writing an introduction to an essay is to inform the reader what he/ she will learn while reading the essay while including the answers to the writing prompt. As a result, your writing will be focused and clear to the reader.

Remember: Think of an introduction to an essay as the paragraph which informs the reader what he/ she will learn in **your** essay as it relates to the topic of the writing prompt

| Introduction: Contains the question I must answer in my essay and the answers I will expand on in your essay. Think what the reader will learn in **your** essay. |

Question: What are the similarities and differences between an apple and an orange?
Answers: Apples and oranges are both fruit that grow on a tree.

Answers: Must be able to expand on your answers as supporting details. You need at least 3 high level answers so that you can provide supporting details

Body Paragraph

What is a body paragraph? A body paragraph has its own main topic sentence and at 3 supporting detail sentences and supports or refers back to the main topic or introduction as it relates to the writing prompt or assignment.

Supporting Detail

What is a supporting detail? Supporting details of a paragraph **explain** the what, where, when, why and how of the main topic or question answered regarding the writing prompt.

How do the supporting details explain or the support the main topic or questions answered in the essay? The following types of information can be used to provide supporting details:

- Explain how something happened and where
- Define words
- Give examples
- State the location, times and dates of events
- Discuss similarities and differences

1. **Body paragraph #1 main topic sentence**:
   Discuss the ***similarities*** between an apple and an orange
   - *Supporting details #1 for body paragraph #1*
     a) Both grow on trees
     b) Both can be eaten peeled
2. **Body paragraph #2 main topic sentence:** The differences between an apple and an orange
   - *Supporting details #2 for body paragraph #2*
     a) An apple's skin can be eaten
     b) An orange's skin can be grated to use ass a zest for a recipe only
3. **Body paragraph #2 main topic sentence:** More differences between an apple and an orange
   - *Supporting details #3 for body paragraph #3*
     a) An orange is easy to share
     b) An orange because it comes pre-sliced from nature

After reviewing the information, I wrote for my body paragraph and supporting details as an outline, I see that will not have enough information or details to write at 3 – 5 sentences as supporting details. I am glad I wrote the outline in an essay format because it helps to focus my writing and helps me to see if I need to develop my details further before I write my essay. Don't worry about the amount of time it takes because the more experience you get with writing the better you will be and the quicker you will get with organizing your thoughts.

Three things:
1. Good, I **wrote** down the outline
2. Good, I wrote down the outline in an essay format
3. Good, I noticed that I need to add more details to my outline before I start writing the essay.

> **Remember** to download the compare and contrast template because it will make writing your compare and contrast outline easier.

Here is my revised supporting detail section for my outline:

Similarities between an apple and an orange
1. Both are fruits
2. Both grow on trees
3. Both can be eaten peeled
4. There are different types of apples and oranges

Differences between an apple and an orange
1. Apple
    a. you can eat the skin
    b. Come in different colors
2. Orange
    a. You can only eat the skin if you grate it and use it as a zest in food
    b. Comes pre-sliced from nature

Conclusion

What is a conclusion? A conclusion does 2 things:

a) Restates the introduction of the essay in different words
b) Informs the reader what he/ she should have learned in the essay

How does the conclusion restate the introduction of the paragraph and inform the reader what he/ she should have learned in the essay? A conclusion can tell the reader what he/ she should have learned in the essay by doing the following:

- Summarizing what the entire essay was about (Hint: use synonyms for the answers to the writing prompt)
- Stating what the reader should know about the main topic as a result of reading the essay

Conclusion: both apples and oranges are fruits, but they are different, if you have pick only one fruit which you may need to share it is easier to share an orange so pick that instead of an apple

This is my final outline. It contains all of the information I need to right a focused 5 paragraph **essay**.

Question: How to learn how to ride a bicycle step-by-step?
Answers: Learn how to balance yourself on the bicycle, learn how to balance yourself and pedal, learn how to stop the bicycle without crashing

Similarities between an apple and an orange
1. Both are fruits
2. Both grow on trees
3. Both can be eaten peeled
4. There are different types of apples and oranges

Differences between an apple and an orange
1. Apple
    a. you can eat the skin
    b. Come in different colors
2. Orange
    a. You can only eat the skin if you grate it and use it as a zest in food
    b. Comes pre-sliced from nature

Conclusion: both apples and oranges are fruits, but they are different, if you have pick only one fruit which you may need to share it is easier to share an orange so pick that instead of an apple

By creating an outline before I start writing my 5 paragraph compare and contrast essay, I can save time, focus my writing and organize my thoughts.

Summary:

Please answer the following questions:

Do you know what an outline is?
Do you know why it is important to write an outline?
Do you know what an introduction is?
Do you know what supporting details are?
Do you know what is a conclusion?

If you answered *no* to any one of the above questions, then re-read entire chapter until you can answer yes to each of the above questions. Why? Because it will help build your knowledge so that when you are faced with the situation of writing a compare and contrast essay, you will know what to do.

If you answered, *yes* to all of the above questions, then we can proceed because you have an action plan in mind of how to write an outline for a 5 paragraph a compare and contrast essay. At the end of the chapter, I will review your knowledge. You can use the information in this chapter to answer the questions so it is open-book, but *you* **must write your answers down.**

Takeaways:

1) An outline is what you are going to write about in an essay or paragraph in list form

2) An outline helps you organize your thoughts list form and helps you see what you are going to write about

3) Supporting details of a paragraph explain the what, where, when, why and how of the main topic or question answered regarding the writing prompt

4) To provide supporting details, you can do the following:
   - Explain how something happened and where
   - Define words
   - Give examples
   - State the location, times and dates of events
   - Discuss similarities and differences

5) A conclusion restates the introduction of the essay in different words and informs the reader what he/ she should have learned in the essay

Review:

Please answer the following questions *in writing or by typing*:

- What is an outline?
- Why it is important to write an outline?
- What is an introduction?
- What are supporting details?
- What is a conclusion?

How do I write my 5 paragraph compare and contrast essay?

In the previous chapter, we learned that an outline can help us organize our thoughts. We are finally going to write the compare and contrast essay using the introduction, 3 body paragraphs with supporting details and conclusion that we created in the outline.

If you need a reminder of the outline we are discussing based on the writing prompt, here it is again:

Question: What are the similarities and differences between an apple and an orange?
Answers: Both are fruits, both grow on trees, both can be eaten peeled, there are different types, you can eat the apple's skin not the orange, orange is easy to share.

Similarities between an apple and an orange

1. Both are fruits
2. Both grow on trees
3. Both can be eaten peeled
4. There are different types of apples and oranges

Differences between an apple and an orange
1. Apple
    a. you can eat the skin
    b. Come in different colors
2. Orange
    a. You can only eat the skin if you grate it and use it as a zest in food
    b. comes pre-sliced from nature

Conclusion: Both apples and oranges are fruits, but they are different, if you have pick only one fruit which you may need to share it is easier to share an orange so pick that instead of an apple.

Now we will write our first draft based on our outline. I will first mention the information from our outline, then I will write the outline in paragraph form for the introduction, body paragraphs and conclusion.

Introduction

From Outline

Question: What are the similarities and differences between an apple and an orange?

Answers: Both are fruits, both grow on trees, both can be eaten peeled, there are different types, you can eat the apple's skin not the orange, orange is easy to share

Outline in paragraph form

What is it like to eat an apple or an orange? Having had eaten both, I can tell you that there are plenty of similarities as well as some differences between an apple and an orange.

Body paragraph # 1 and Supporting details for it

From Outline

Similarities between an apple and an orange
1. Both are fruits
2. Both grow on trees
3. Both can be eaten peeled
4. There are different types of apples and oranges

Outline in paragraph form

First, an apple and an orange both have many traits in common. For instance, both grow on trees. They both can be eaten peeled and there are different types of each. An apple is a granny smith or a gala apple. An orange is a navel orange or a regular orange.

Body paragraph # 2 and Supporting details for it

From Outline

1) You can eat the skin of an apple, not an orange

Outline in paragraph form

Next, there are big differences between an apple and an orange. For instance, the skin of an apple can be eaten, but not an orange unless you want to get sick. The only way the skin of an orange can be eaten is if it is grated and used as zest for a meal.

Body paragraph # 3 and Supporting detail #3

From Outline

4) An orange is easier to share than an apple
   a) Orange pre-sliced
   b) Must cut an apple with a knife to have slices

© http://www.beststudentsuccessseries.com

Outline in paragraph form

Third, an orange is more convenient to eat especially if you have to share. Although you can slice an apple with a knife, if you want to share it. An orange is easier to share because it is already pre-sliced once you peel the skin off.

Conclusion

From Outline

    An orange is easier to share than an apple

Outline in paragraph form

In conclusion, an apple and an orange are both fruits, but they are different. If you have to pick one fruit over the other and there is a possibility that you may need to share it, then it is better to pick an orange because it is easier to share than an apple.

Here is my **final** draft of my essay:

What is it like to eat an apple or an orange? Having had eaten both, I can tell you that there are plenty of similarities as well as some differences between an apple and an orange.

First, an apple and an orange both have many traits in common. For instance, both grow on trees. They both can be eaten peeled and there are different types of each. An apple is a granny smith or a gala apple. An orange is a navel orange or a regular orange.

Next, there are big differences between an apple and an orange. For instance, the skin of an apple can be eaten, but not an orange unless you want to get sick. The only way the skin of an orange can be eaten is if it is grated and used as zest for a meal.

Third, an orange is more convenient to eat especially if you have to share. Although you can slice an apple with a knife, if you want to share it. An orange is easier to share because it is already pre-sliced once you peel the skin off.

In conclusion, an apple and an orange are both fruits, but they are different. If you have to pick one fruit over the other and there is a possibility that you may need to share it, then it is better to pick an orange because it is easier to share than an apple.

Summary:

Please answer the following questions:

Do you understand how to write a clear, concise 5 paragraph compare and contrast essay now?

Do you understand how to put it together from understanding the writing prompt so that you answer the right questions?

Do you understand how to write and/ or rewrite a quick outline to map out or layout your thoughts in a clear, concise manner?

Do you understand how to write your outline in paragraph form for the introduction, 3 body paragraphs, and conclusion?

If you answered, *no* to any one of the above questions, then re-read all the entire chapter until you can answer yes to each of the above questions. Why? Because it will help build your knowledge so that when you are faced with the situation of writing an explanatory essay, you will know what to do.

If you answered, *yes* to all of the above questions, then we can proceed because you have an action plan in mind of how to write a 5 paragraph explanatory essay. At the end of the chapter, I will review your knowledge. You can use the information in this chapter to answer the questions so it is open-book, but *you* **must** write your answers down.

Takeaways:

1) Use keywords to identify what type of essay you need to write
2) Turn your writing prompt into a question to focus your writing
3) Pre-writing or brainstorming will help organize your thoughts and clear your mind to focus your writing
4) Writing an outline can help you organize your thoughts
5) Use your outline to write your essay in paragraph form

Review:

Please answer the following questions *in writing or by typing*:
- How do you understand a writing prompt?
- What is pre-writing?
- What is the purpose of an outline?

Lessons Learned

Now that you have learned the system to write a 5 paragraph explanatory essay, I hope that you found this book easy to understand. Do you understand that writing is a process and your final essay may look different at different stages? Do you feel that you learned how to write a 5 paragraph explanatory essay? I hope your answer is yes. Do you think you will use the book as a reference? I hope your answer is yes.

I Know How to Write a Compare and Contrast Essay, Now What?

In order to improve your writing even further, I want you to do the following:
1. Read writing assignments carefully to make sure that you answer every point
2. Re-read your essay yourself before showing it to anyone so that you can make sure it sounds like you want even I have to do this
3. Get assignments competed earlier than the deadline, if possible. Why? Then, you can ask your teacher advice on how to improve your writing before the due date

I recommend that you look at this book as a good starting point and read my other books too.

Next, please go to my website which is beststudentsuccessseries.com. It offers more writing courses and points you to references which will help you improve your writing.

I shared with you my system on writing a 5 paragraph explanatory essay. It helped me to learn how to improve my writing and as a result I started speaking more clearly. I hope that you notice the same in yourself.

I would like to hear from you. Please your comments about your results on amazon.com and on my website.

Appendix A - Transition Words

Transition words help control the flow as a person writes or reads from paragraph to paragraph to make it clear as well as smooth. Here are a few transitions you can use.

- in the first place
- not only ... but also
- as a matter of fact
- in like manner
- in addition
- coupled with
- in the same fashion / way
- first, second, third
- in the light of
- not to mention
- to say nothing of
- equally important
- by the same token
- again
- to
- and
- also
- then
- equally
- identically
- uniquely
- like
- as
- too
- moreover
- as well as
- together with
- of course
- likewise
- comparatively
- correspondingly
- similarly
- furthermore
- additionally

www.ingramcontent.com/pod-product-compliance
Lightning Source LLC
Chambersburg PA
CBHW070735230426
43665CB00016B/2255